FELDENKRAIS METHOD

The Complete Guide To Feldenkrais Method: Understanding The Tradition, Technique, And Transformative Healing

BANABAS WISDOM

Contents

Introductory

By increasing self-awareness through movement, the Feldenkrais Method is a somatic educational approach that seeks to improve movement and physical function.

Individuals can improve their physical and mental health by developing a greater awareness of their movements and by learning new ways to move, according to the premise underlying this technique.

The technique consists of a sequence of slow, delicate movements that are intentionally executed to heighten awareness of ingrained movement patterns and investigate novel potentialities for effortless and effective motion.

Two Primary Elements Comprise The Feldenkrais Method:

• Awareness Through Movement (ATM): This course consists of group instruction in which an instructor leads students through a series of movements while encouraging them to consider alternative methods of carrying out familiar actions. Increasing awareness of the body's movements, sensations, and the interrelationships among its various elements is the primary objective.

• Functional Integration (FI): This is a one-on-one approach in which a Feldenkrais practitioner guides an individual through personalized movements through the use of verbal prompts and gentle touch.

In addition to addressing specific movement patterns or limitations, the objective is to assist the individual in discovering more comfortable and efficient methods of movement.

The Feldenkrais Method is implemented to enhance balance,

flexibility, coordination, and posture, among other qualities. Individuals who are recovering from injuries, seeking alleviation from chronic pain, or aiming to improve their overall well-being frequently utilize it.

The Feldenkrais Method is characterized by its focus on mindful movement and heightened self-awareness, which sets it apart from conventional exercise or physical therapy methodologies.

CHAPTER ONE
The Relationship Between The Mind And Body In Feldenkrais

Aware that our physical movements are intricately linked to our mental and emotional states, the Feldenkrais Method places considerable emphasis on the mind-body connection. Key elements of the Feldenkrais Method's mind-body connection include the following:

• The Feldenkrais Method is predicated on the notion that heightened consciousness of one's movements can result in enhanced physical functionality and overall welfare. Through deliberate awareness of bodily sensations and movement quality, people can acquire self-awareness regarding their patterns of behavior, develop more efficient motor skills, and alleviate superfluous muscular strain.

• The method promotes the practice of mindful exploration when considering potential movements. By employing subtle and delicate motions, practitioners direct individuals to investigate a variety of motion patterns.

This investigation encompasses not only tangible behaviors but also an intensified cognizance of the emotions, thoughts, and sensations linked to said movements.

- The Feldenkrais Method is founded upon the principle of neuroplasticity, which refers to the capacity of the brain to undergo structural reorganization as a result of personal experience.

Through deliberate and inventive motion patterns, people have the ability to generate fresh neural connections, which in turn facilitates enhanced motor control and coordination. Those afflicted with pain, ailments, or limitations in movement may find this especially beneficial.

• Emotional and psychological well-being are encompassed within Feldenkrais' mind-body connection, which extends beyond physical movements.

As people increase their self-awareness regarding their bodies and movement patterns, they may also observe correlations between their emotional states and physical behaviors. Developing an awareness of and adjusting to these patterns may enhance one's emotional health.

• Feldenkrais places significant emphasis on the concept of "effortless action," which entails the execution of movements with minimal superfluous strain and exertion. Mental and physical stress and tension can be alleviated through the development of a sense of comfort in movement.

• The primary objective of the Feldenkrais Method is to achieve a state of harmonious integration between the body and psyche. As a method of self-improvement and self-discovery, movement enables people to gain a deeper comprehension of themselves and their capacity for transformation.

The Feldenkrais Method advocates for a comprehensive approach to movement education, recognizing the intrinsic interdependence of the physical and mental spheres. By cultivating heightened consciousness and doing introspective inquiry, people have the capacity to improve their physical, emotional, and cognitive welfare.

Fundamental Tenets Of Feldenkrais

The Feldenkrais Method is founded upon a set of foundational principles that dictate its methodology for movement instruction and enhancement. Listed below are some fundamental tenets of the Feldenkrais Method:

• Awareness: The notion of awareness is fundamental to the Feldenkrais Method. Recognizing and valuing the quality of one's movements, patterns, and overall movement awareness is regarded as crucial for the purposes of learning and development.

By cultivating mindful attention, people have the ability to uncover more comfortable and effective methods of movement.

• In general, the Feldenkrais Method employs movements that are gradual, non-intrusive, and gentle. The primary focus is on investigating motions that require the least amount of exertion, enabling people to maintain their ease of motion and circumvent superfluous tension.

• Exploration and variation are fostered in movement patterns through the implementation of this method. Through the practice of performing familiar actions in various variations, people have the ability to broaden their repertoire of movements and uncover novel opportunities for effortless and effective motion.

• Observation without prejudice: Non-judgmental observation is emphasized. By encouraging participants to observe and investigate their movements without ascribing labels of "correct" or "incorrect," an environment conducive to open and constructive learning is fostered devoid of prejudice.

- Movements utilizing the Feldenkrais Method frequently entail nuanced and minor modifications. By attending to subtle alterations and sensations, people can develop a more refined awareness and a more precise sense of motor control.

- Functional Integration (FI) entails individualized sessions during which practitioners employ verbal guidance and gentle contact to assist clients in exploring movement patterns. This individualized methodology facilitates a heightened level of consciousness and customized investigation in accordance with the specific requirements of each person.

• The Feldenkrais Method is founded on the notion that the brain is capable of undergoing modifications and adjustments in response to experience. Through the practice of innovative and mindful movements, people have the ability to develop fresh neural pathways and enhance their overall movement patterns.

• Overall Body Engagement: The approach frequently emphasizes movements that encompass the entire body, as opposed to isolating particular muscles or body regions. This holistic approach advocates for coordinated, integrated movement by acknowledging the interdependence of bodily systems.

• The Feldenkrais Method promotes the investigation of "effortless action," which entails identifying techniques for executing movements with reduced strain and effort, thereby facilitating enhanced efficiency and comfort.

• Functional development is the overarching objective of the Feldenkrais Method. Its execution aims to augment an individual's capacity to carry out routine tasks with increased flexibility, comfort, and ease.

The amalgamation of these principles in the Feldenkrais Method results in a distinctive and comprehensive approach that renders it a valuable instrument for enhancing motor function, alleviating discomfort, and fostering general welfare.

CHAPTER TWO
Investigating Awareness Via Movement Instruction

Lessons in "Awareness Through Movement" (ATM) are an essential element of the Feldenkrais Method. Lessons are commonly delivered in collaborative environments, either via live instruction or pre-recorded audio lectures.

The objective of ATM lessons is to direct individuals through a sequence of movements, thereby cultivating heightened consciousness of their ingrained patterns and investigating novel potentialities for motion.

Consider the following factors when investigating Awareness Through Movement lessons:

• Concentrate on the nature of your experience, your sensations, and your movements as you practice mindful attention. The primary focus is on fostering consciousness as opposed to attaining precise results. Observe the various body regions that are engaged in the movements.

• Generally, the movements performed in ATM courses are slow and gentle. This enables heightened consciousness and responsiveness to nuanced alterations. Avoid forcing yourself into discomfort; for ease of movement, prioritize simplicity over exertion.

• Exploration and Variation: The courses frequently incorporate inventive renditions of routine movements. Appraise these variations with inquisitiveness and a receptive mindset. This can assist in breaking down routines and broadening one's repertoire of movements.

• Adopt a non-judgmental stance when observing the movements. A "correct" or "incorrect" method of movement does not exist according to Feldenkrais. Rather, observe your natural movement and remain receptive to the possibility of discovering more efficient alternatives.

• Breathing Awareness: Throughout the movements, pay close attention to your respiration. Lessons frequently incorporate breathing exercises as a means to augment general consciousness and promote relaxation. Observe the correlation between your respiration and various movements.

• The integration of the body and psyche entails acknowledging their inherent interdependence. The Feldenkrais Method advocates for the utilization of movement as a vehicle for self-exploration and enhancement, fostering a comprehensive comprehension of the individual.

• Integration and Rest: Certain classes might incorporate intervals of stillness or repose. Leverage these intervals to synthesize the perceptions and understandings acquired while in motion. The inclusion of this reflective element is vital to the learning process.

• Regular practice and consistency are factors that can augment the advantages of ATM lessons. Consistent practice facilitates continuous improvement and exploration of one's movement. Over time, you might discover that your awareness and movement patterns change.

• Adjust for Comfort: In the event that a particular motion causes discomfort or pain, adjust it accordingly to align with your preferred level of comfort. Comfort and flexibility are of the utmost importance to the Feldenkrais Method, and practitioners are encouraged to modify their movements to suit their specific requirements.

• Feel free to share your experiences and ask questions when participating in a group class led by a teacher or facilitator; this promotes open communication. Instructors may utilize verbal signals to direct students' attention and offer guidance regarding potential movements.

Bear in mind that the experience of each individual with Awareness Through Movement teachings is distinct. Self-improvement and self-discovery comprise the process, which has no predetermined conclusion. By adopting an attitude of inquisitiveness, receptiveness, and conscious awareness during the lessons, one can acquire significant knowledge regarding their movement patterns and potentially uncover more streamlined and comfortable techniques of motion.

Practical Instruction In Functional Integration

The practical component of the Feldenkrais Method, Functional Integration (FI) serves as a supplement to the collective instruction of Awareness Through Movement (ATM).

A trained Feldenkrais practitioner works individually with a pupil during FI sessions, guiding them through new possibilities for efficient and comfortable movement through the use of verbal guidance and gentle touch.

Key elements to keep in mind regarding Functional Integration hands-on sessions are as follows:

- Tailored Approach: FI sessions are exceptionally individualized and constructed to address the particular concerns and requirements of each participant. By observing the client's posture, movements, and general organization, the practitioner develops individualized interventions.

- Practitioners employ the technique of gentle contact as a method of communication. The purpose of the non-intrusive contact is to stimulate the nervous system with feedback, thereby increasing awareness of the body's movement organization.

- Verbal guidance is an additional modality employed by practitioners to augment the client's awareness, alongside physical contact. This may encompass signals that direct attention towards particular sensations, movements, or imagery, all of which contribute to a more comfortable and efficient mode of movement.

- Exploration of Movements: The practitioner conducts the client through a series of movements, which are frequently subtle and small, in order to investigate various patterns and possibilities. The primary focus is on movement quality and identifying methods to minimize superfluous exertion and tension.

• Enhanced Sensory Awareness: FI sessions strive to augment the client's sensory awareness by employing a blend of tactile stimulation and verbal instructions. A greater level of consciousness can result in beneficial modifications to one's posture, movement patterns, and overall functionality.

• Integration of Body and Mind: FI sessions, similar to ATM teachings, acknowledge the interdependence of the body and mind. The experiential learning is intended to cultivate a comprehensive comprehension of one's self, encouraging constructive transformations in mental and emotional health as well as physical mobility.

• Ensuring the comfort and wellbeing of the client is of the utmost importance. Practitioners are instructed to operate within the boundaries of the client's comfort zone, and effective communication between the practitioner and the client is promoted to guarantee a constructive and positive session.

• FI sessions have the capacity to be modified in order to facilitate participants who have a range of physical conditions or limitations. It is possible to tailor the method to the specific requirements of each individual client.

• FI sessions provide an occasion for individuals to engage in self-discovery. Frequently, clients acquire awareness regarding their bodily movements and discover methods to alleviate superfluous stress, resulting in enhanced overall functionality and welfare.

• In contrast to the self-directed investigation emphasized in ATM lessons, FI sessions offer a more structured and guided experience. Collective instruction and practical application—both elements—are mutually reinforcing in their ability to provide a holistic approach to movement education.

Functional Integration is frequently pursued for a multitude of motives, encompassing but not limited to pain alleviation, enhanced mobility, and improved activity performance.

Working with a certified Feldenkrais practitioner is advised in order to fully benefit from Functional Integration sessions.

CHAPTER THREE
Practical Feldenkrais Techniques

To incorporate the tenets of the Feldenkrais Method into one's daily life, it is necessary to incorporate mindfulness, movement exploration, and consciousness into routine tasks. The following are some suggestions for integrating Feldenkrais principles into one's daily life:

1. Engaging in Mindful Movement During Routine Activities:

• It is imperative to be mindful of one's movement while performing everyday tasks such as standing, walking, reclining, and reaching.

• It is advisable to cultivate an awareness of one's posture and experiment with different variations in order to discover more comfortable and effective methods of movement.

2. Breathing Observance:

• Develop a heightened awareness of your respiration, particularly when experiencing stress or tension.

• Observe the impact that your natural and effortless breathing has on your overall state of wellness.

3. Implementing Effortless Action:

• To optimize performance, adopt the mindset of "effortless action." Contemplate methods to carry out duties with minimal superfluous exertion and strain.

4. Investigation into Movement Variations:

• One may engage in experimentation by executing familiar actions in various methods. Alternate your walking cadence, for instance, and consider alternative sitting and standing positions.

• Please take note of the substantial impact that minor adjustments can have on comfort and mobility.

5. Scan of the Body and Relaxation:

• Scan your body periodically for areas of tension. Forcefully alleviate tension and promote a state of serenity.

• Incorporate brief intervals of stretching or moderate movement into your daily routine to mitigate the negative effects of extended periods of sitting or performing repetitive duties.

6. Precautions Regarding Commuting:

• It is imperative to maintain physical and mental awareness during one's commute, whether it be by foot, automobile, or public transportation.

- During this period, investigate nuanced motions, such as making a slight head turn or modifying your seating position.

7. Sensory Consciousness:

- Develop sensory awareness by directing your attention towards the bodily sensations that accompany your movements.

Investigate the textures of surfaces beneath your soles, the sensation of air on your skin, and the motion of your clothing.

8. The incorporation of exercise routines:

• To incorporate Feldenkrais's principles into one's exercise regimen, prioritize the quality of movements over their quantity.

• Investigate the use of exercise variations as a means to augment flexibility, coordination, and holistic body consciousness.

9. Practicing Mindful Eating:

• Raise your awareness regarding your eating habits. Observe the bodily actions associated with food retrieval, elevation, and entry into the mouth.

• One should contemplate different ways to hold implements or sit at the table in order to facilitate comfort and ease.

10. Reflect and Acquire Knowledge:

• Consider the experiences that have transpired during the course of the day. Observe any modifications to your gait, level of comfort, and general state of being.

• Leverage this heightened self-awareness to direct your investigation into movement patterns during subsequent endeavors.

The integration of Feldenkrais principles into one's daily existence necessitates a steadfast dedication to continuous exploration and mindful awareness.

The objective is to optimize one's general state of health by cultivating a more profound equilibrium between the physical and mental faculties and uncovering more streamlined and pleasant methods of locomotion. Curiousness and consistent practice in daily activities can result in gradual positive changes.

Feldenkrais's Approach To Particular Populations

The Feldenkrais Method is renowned for its adaptability and potential to provide benefits to diverse populations, including individuals confronted with particular obstacles or circumstances.

The subsequent instances illustrate the application of Feldenkrais to particular populations:

1. Athletes and entertainers:

• Feldenkrais can be utilized to optimize athletic performance through the development of increased coordination, flexibility, and movement efficacy.

• One way in which it can aid in injury prevention is through the instruction of athletes on how to move with increased fluidity and decreased effort.

2. Chronic Musculoskeletal Disorders and Pain:

• Individuals who are afflicted with musculoskeletal disorders or chronic discomfort may discover alleviation via Feldenkrais.

• The approach prioritizes mindful and gentle motions, enabling people to experiment with novel motions that alleviate tension and discomfort.

3. Disorders of the nervous system (such as multiple sclerosis and stroke):

• Feldenkrais can be modified to enhance mobility and coordination in individuals with neurological conditions.

• The method's emphasis on neuroplasticity is especially pertinent for individuals who are interested in improving the connections between the brain and body following neurological impairments.

4. Disabilities in Learning and Children:

• Feldenkrais can improve coordination and body awareness in children with cognitive disabilities, which are both advantageous outcomes.

• The method's exploratory and patient approach may captivate children, facilitating the development of a more comfortable and efficient gait.

5. An aging populace:

• Feldenkrais can assist the elderly in preserving or enhancing their balance, mobility, and overall functionality.

• Owing to its focus on flexibility and personalized instruction, the approach is highly suitable for attending to the distinct requirements of elderly individuals.

6. Stress and Anxiety:

• Anxiety and tension sufferers may benefit from Feldenkrais's techniques, which encourage mindfulness and relaxation.

- Promoting a state of tranquility and enhancing one's general state of health can be accomplished through the utilization of mindful breathing and composed movements.

7. Rehabilitation following an operation or trauma:

- Feldenkrais can serve as a supplementary modality to rehabilitation following surgery or injury through the encouragement of controlled and mild movements.

- It has the potential to facilitate the restoration of functional movement patterns and mitigate the development of compensatory behaviors that might arise throughout the recovery process.

8. Regarding Ergonomics and Posture:

• Individuals who experience distress or posture-related issues as a result of extended sitting can derive advantages from Feldenkrais.

• The approach promotes the examination of one's postural practices and the development of more ergonomic positions for sitting, standing, and motion.

9. Well-being of the Emotions and Mindfulness:

- Feldenkrais's integration of the body-mind connection confers advantages to practitioners who are interested in cultivating emotional well-being and mindfulness.

- Additionally, the method's emphasis on mindful movement and self-awareness may aid in tension reduction and enhanced concentration.

10. Individuals with Movement Restrictions:

- Fieldenkrais can be modified to accommodate individuals who have physical disabilities or restrictions on their movement.

- The method's emphasis on exploratory, small-scale movements facilitates a progressive and flexible strategy for enhancing overall functionality.

It is crucial to emphasize that although Feldenkrais may offer advantages for numerous populations, it should not be considered a replacement for therapeutic or medical interventions. It is advisable for individuals with particular health concerns to seek guidance from healthcare professionals prior to commencing any novel exercise regimen or movement routine.

Certified Feldenkrais practitioners possess the ability to offer individualized consultations and modify the approach in order to accommodate the requirements of heterogeneous populations.

CHAPTER FOUR
The Method As An Intersection Of Mindfulness

Both the Feldenkrais Method and mindfulness place equal importance on the interplay between the mind and body, as well as on awareness and presence. The following is an examination of how mindfulness and the Feldenkrais Method intersect:

1. Presence and Awareness:

• Both mindfulness and the Feldenkrais Method prioritize the development of mindfulness and the state of being fully present in the present moment. The aforementioned practices promote the non-judgmental observation of one's thoughts, sensations, and movements.

2. Mind-Body Interaction:

• Both approaches acknowledge the profound interdependence of the mind and body. It is recognized that mental states have the potential to impact physical health, and conversely. An effort is made to harmonize the body and mind in pursuit of holistic health.

3. Non-Evaluative Observation:

• Mindfulness promotes the practice of impartially observing one's thoughts and sensations. In a similar vein, the Feldenkrais Method encourages a critical examination of movement, permitting individuals to observe and acquire knowledge without ascribing moral or immoral standards.

4. Investigationism and Inquisitiveness:

• Both mindfulness and the Feldenkrais Method are characterized by an inventive and inquisitive spirit. Exploring movement possibilities in Feldenkrais and contemplating thoughts and emotions in mindfulness both encourage individuals to be inquisitive about their experiences.

5. Patience and Gentleness:

• Both practices place significant emphasis on the virtues of forbearance and gentleness. A compassionate and patient disposition toward one's thoughts and emotions is fostered by mindfulness. The Feldenkrais Method encourages the use of delicate movements, refraining from the application of force or strain.

6. Breath Observation:

• Mindfulness frequently integrates the awareness of one's respiration as a central focus of attention. Likewise, breath awareness is frequently incorporated into movement courses as a means to augment general awareness and relaxation, as advocated by the Feldenkrais Method.

7. Sensory Consciousness:

• The Feldenkrais Method and mindfulness both require heightened sensory awareness. Engaging in Feldenkrais's exploration of subtle movements or mindfulness's attention to bodily sensations both encourage individuals to be completely present with their sensory experiences.

8. The incorporation of daily life:

• The practice of mindfulness is frequently implemented in everyday life to heighten awareness of mundane tasks. In a similar fashion, the Feldenkrais Method promotes the incorporation of enhanced movement patterns into one's everyday life, thereby cultivating an ongoing consciousness of one's own movements.

9. Body-Mind Resilience:

• Both of these practices enhance mental and physical resilience. The Feldenkrais Method can improve physical resilience by encouraging adaptable and efficient movement patterns, while mindfulness can enhance mental resilience.

10.   **Self-Exploration and Development:**

- Both mindfulness and the Feldenkrais Method facilitate individual development and self-discovery. By cultivating introspection and investigation, people may discover fresh perspectives regarding themselves and their capacity to effect constructive transformation.

Although mindfulness and the Feldenkrais Method are separate practices, their common principles enhance our comprehension of the interplay between the body and mind. It is possible that individuals will discover that integrating both methodologies into their daily lives results in improved holistic health, heightened self-awareness, and an enhanced capacity to confront everyday obstacles.

Feldenkrais And Reinforcement

In numerous rehabilitation contexts, the Feldenkrais Method has been utilized to aid patients recovering from surgeries, injuries, and chronic conditions. Feldenkrais can provide the following benefits to the rehabilitation process:

1. Increased Physical Awareness:

- A heightened awareness of one's physique and movement patterns is fostered by Feldenkrais. Enhanced self-awareness can prove to be highly advantageous in the context of rehabilitation, as it enables participants to identify and confront compensatory behaviors or routines that may have emerged throughout the course of recovery.

2. Adaptive and Mild Motions:

- The approach employs mild and flexible motions, rendering it appropriate for individuals at different phases of the rehabilitation process. Rebuilding movement patterns is accomplished in a gradual and non-intrusive manner through the emphasis on patient exploration.

3. Extension of Range of Motion:

• Feldenkrais courses frequently encompass an extensive repertoire of movements with the aim of enhancing joint mobility and flexibility. Individuals recuperating from surgeries or injuries that have restricted their range of motion may find this to be advantageous.

4. Rehabilitation and Neuroplasticity:

• Based on the principle of neuroplasticity, which is the brain's capacity to reorganize itself, The Feldenkrais Method was developed. Through the practice of deliberate and unique motions, people have the ability to energize neural pathways, thereby facilitating the restoration of motor control and coordination.

5. Muscle Tension and Pain Reduction:

• Numerous individuals undergoing rehabilitation suffer from muscle tension and discomfort. The implementation of Feldenkrais lessons, which prioritize the release of superfluous muscular tension, has the potential to alleviate pain and distress.

6. Posture and Alignment Improvements:

• Feldenkrais places emphasis on the enhancement of posture and overall body alignment. Particularly advantageous for those recuperating from surgeries or injuries that may have altered their posture.

7. Individualized Methodology:

• Feldenkrais practitioners customize sessions to address the unique requirements of every participant. By employing a personalized approach, movements can be modified to suit the specific needs and objectives of the individual undergoing rehabilitation.

8. Enhanced Balance and Coordination:

• The objective of the method is to enhance balance and coordination by means of mindful movement exploration. This is beneficial for patients who are in the process of recuperating from conditions that could have affected their balance or motor coordination.

9. Harmonization of the Body and Mind:

• The Feldenkrais Method acknowledges the interdependence of physical and mental health by integrating the mind and body. Adopting a holistic approach has the potential to enhance an individual's holistic recovery and well-being.

10. Biological Complement to Other Therapies:

• Feldenkrais' methods have the potential to supplement conventional rehabilitation modalities, including occupational therapy and physical therapy. By providing a distinct viewpoint on movement and self-awareness, it augments the efficacy of a rehabilitation program that integrates multiple disciplines.

It is imperative that individuals undergoing rehabilitation seek the advice of their healthcare providers prior to implementing any novel movement regimen.

Healthcare professionals can collaborate with certified Feldenkrais practitioners who possess expertise in rehabilitation to deliver sessions that are adaptable and supportive, with a focus on the unique requirements of the individual undergoing recovery.

CHAPTER FIVE
Feldenkrais In Well-Being And Creativity

An investigation has been conducted into the Feldenkrais Method as a means of augmenting creativity and general welfare. Feldenkrais can make the following contributions to the following facets of the human experience:

1. Enhanced Physical Awareness:

• A heightened awareness of bodily sensations and movements is emphasized by Feldenkrais. This heightened consciousness may affect an individual's mental and emotional state as well, thereby promoting a more profound comprehension of oneself.

2. Alleviation of Stress and Tension:

• Feldenkrais movements, by their exploratory and non-violent character, have the potential to facilitate the alleviation of physical tension and stress. An equanimous state of mind may accompany a heightened state of physical relaxation.

3. Enhanced Response to Relaxation:

• Feldenkrais promotes a parasympathetic nervous system response, also known as relaxation. This practice may engender favorable impacts on one's mental health by fostering a state of tranquility and repose.

4. Practice of mindfulness and presence:

• The approach integrates principles of mindfulness, encouraging participants to remain entirely present and invested in the investigation of bodily movements.

Engaging in other facets of life while cultivating a sense of presence and mindfulness is possible.

5. The Promotion of Neuroplasticity:

• Feldenkrais's approach is founded upon the principle of neuroplasticity, which pertains to the capacity of the brain to undergo self-reorganization. Possible benefits of engaging in mindful and novel movements include the stimulation of neural pathways, which may increase cognitive function and creativity.

6. Investigation of Movement Potentialities:

• Feldenkrais courses promote the exploration of an extensive array of movement possibilities among participants. This investigation may provoke an attitude of inquisitiveness and receptiveness, which in turn encourages innovative thought and problem-solving.

7. Posture and Alignment Improvements:

• Optimal body alignment and equilibrium have the potential to exert a beneficial impact on mental and emotional states. Enhanced posture and alignment facilitated by Feldenkrais may positively impact an individual's confidence and sense of well-being.

8. Comprehensive Body Integration:

• Feldenkrais considers the body to be an interconnected, whole system. Adopting a holistic perspective can motivate people to evaluate their overall health and wellness by taking into account physical, mental, and emotional dimensions.

9. Adaptability in Thought:

• Movement exploration promotes adaptability and flexibility, which can be extrapolated to enhance mental flexibility as well. This can be advantageous in cultivating innovative thinking and the capacity to tackle obstacles from various vantage points.

10. The incorporation of daily life:

• This integration promotes a way of life in which self-care and mindfulness are given precedence.

11. Emotional Communication:

• Frequently, movement is associated with emotional expression. Feldenkrais can facilitate the exploration and expression of emotions through non-verbal means, thereby promoting emotional well-being.

12. Reduction of Stress and Resilience:

• Feldenkrais's advocacy for relaxation and tension reduction may ultimately foster increased resilience when confronted with the trials and tribulations of life. Consequently, this can have a beneficial effect on one's general state of well-being.

Although Feldenkrais cannot replace interventions that specifically target mental health or creativity, it can serve as a beneficial supplement to a comprehensive approach to overall well-being. A significant number of people discover that the technique improves their quality of life by encouraging mindfulness, physical comfort, and a sense of exploration and ingenuity.

Common Obstacles Encountered In Feldenkrais Practice

Although employing the Feldenkrais Method can yield significant benefits, there are specific challenges that individuals may confront. The following are several prevalent obstacles and prospective approaches to overcome them:

1. Persistence and Patience:

• Obstacle: The rate of progress in Feldenkrais may be incremental, and certain individuals might discover it difficult to maintain a persistent and patient approach to their practice.

• Approach: Embrace the process
and recognize incremental progress.
Establish reasonable objectives and
perceive the practice as an ongoing
process rather than a final product.

2. The process of self-judgment:

• One potential challenge is that
individuals might be susceptible to
self-criticism or frustration when
they perceive their actions as lacking
effectiveness or as "wrong."

• One approach is to develop a non-
judgmental disposition. Bear in
mind that the objective of
Feldenkrais is exploration, not
perfection. Placing emphasis on the

process of learning rather than attaining a particular result is crucial.

3. Opposition to Change:

• Certain individuals might be resistant to experimenting with novel movement patterns or altering established routines.

• Approach the practice with an attitude of inquiry and receptiveness. Exhibit a readiness to investigate and accept the possibility of constructive transformation.

4. Intense discomfort or pain:

• One challenge is that certain conditions may cause distress for individuals during physical activity, which may result in avoidance behavior.

• Approach: Engage in candid dialogue with a Feldenkrais practitioner regarding any feelings of unease. Frequently, movements can be modified to accommodate specific requirements. Prioritizing comfort and avoiding painful movements are both essential.

5. Challenges with assimilating into everyday life:

• Difficulty may be encountered by some individuals in applying Feldenkrais principles to their daily lives.

• To begin, implement a methodical and incremental modification to your daily movements. With perseverance and regularity, systematically incorporate Feldenkrais principles into diverse facets of your daily regimen.

6. Contemplating Time for Practice:

• Obstacles may find it difficult to allocate specific time for Feldenkrais practice due to their hectic schedules.

• To achieve this, integrate brief, meditative movements into one's daily routine. The importance of consistency outweighs that of each practice session's extent. Consider enrolling in group classes or utilizing online resources to obtain structured instruction.

7. Sensory Deluge:

• Obstacle: Certain individuals may perceive the simultaneous attention to movements and sensations as excessive, particularly if they lack experience with such a heightened state of awareness.

• Strategy: Commence with basic movements and progressively elevate their intricacy. Take necessary pauses. Sensory awareness will develop into a more natural state over time.

8. Restricted Access to Courses:

• One potential obstacle is the potential scarcity of certified

Feldenkrais practitioners or classes in specific areas.

• One potential approach is to investigate digital resources, such as audio recordings or video lectures. Although in-person seminars provide individualized instruction, online resources can be extremely beneficial for self-study.

9. The Assemblage of Mindfulness:

• One possible challenge for individuals who are not well-versed in mindfulness practices is the integration of Feldenkrais's mindfulness component, which requires complete presence and awareness.

• To commence, adopt a basic respiration awareness technique. Lend this state of mindfulness to movements gradually. Permit yourself to be completely present, judgment-free, in each moment.

10. Locating an Appropriate Instructor:

• One potential challenge is the existence of divergent personal preferences regarding instruction styles, which could result in a prolonged search for a Feldenkrais practitioner whose methodology aligns with your own.

Attend classes taught by a variety of practitioners and be receptive to experimenting with various teaching techniques. It is critical to find a practitioner with whom you have a good rapport in order to have a positive experience.

Bear in mind that each individual's Feldenkrais voyage is distinct, and that difficulties are an inherent aspect of the learning process. By cultivating open communication with a certified Feldenkrais practitioner, adopting self-compassion, and demonstrating a willingness to investigate, it is possible to surmount these challenges and optimize the method's benefits.

Summary

The Feldenkrais Method provides an exceptional and comprehensive approach to movement education and overall health. Based on the foundational tenets of consciousness, flexibility, and the interrelation between the mind and body, Feldenkrais offers a structured approach to examining and enhancing motor patterns.

The method promotes the cultivation of a more profound self-awareness and capability for constructive transformation, whether it be in the context of rehabilitation, creativity, or everyday existence.

Through the promotion of mindfulness, facilitation of tactful inquiry, and prioritization of flexibility, Feldenkrais aids people in the revelation of more optimal and comfortable motions. Consequently, this can lead to improvements in physical comfort, emotional welfare, and overall life satisfaction.

Although there may be obstacles to overcome, including impatience, self-criticism, and the integration of the practice into one's daily routine, these challenges present prospects for personal development. A nonjudgmental attitude, perseverance, and patience are essential for navigating the learning process.

Feldenkrais's applicability spans across diverse populations, encompassing athletes, individuals managing chronic conditions, those undergoing rehabilitation, and those aiming to augment their creative capabilities. By incorporating mindfulness, neuroplasticity, and a whole-body approach, the method distinguishes itself as a multifunctional and advantageous instrument for personal growth and exploration.

In essence, the Feldenkrais Method encourages people to engage in an exploratory process, recognizing the capacity for constructive transformations in their physicality, mentality, and general state of being.

By engaging in Feldenkrais techniques, whether independently or under the supervision of a certified practitioner, one can attain a more attuned and harmonious connection between the physical and mental realms.

THE END